The Complete Lean & Green Cookbook

Easy And Healthy Lean & Green Recipes For Weight Loss

Jesse Cohen

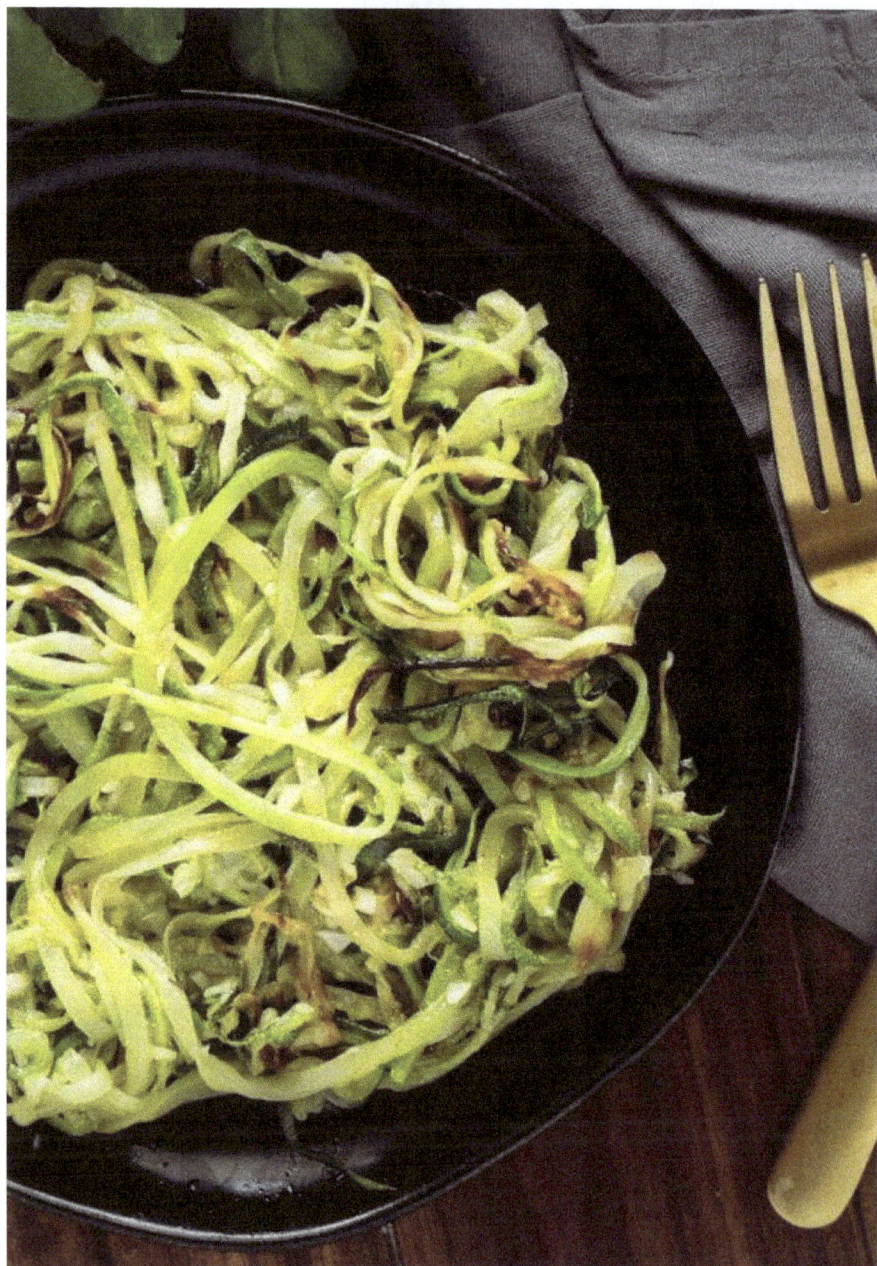

Table of contents

Chicken, Kale & Cucumber Salad

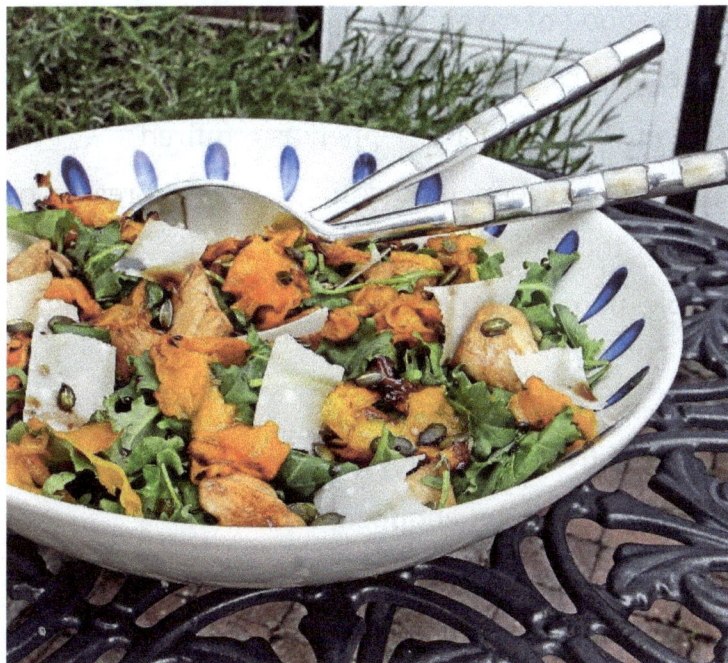

Servings: 4

Preparation Time: 15 minutes

Cooking Time: 18 minutes

Ingredients:

For Chicken:

- 1 teaspoon of dried thyme

- ½ teaspoon of garlic powder
- ½ teaspoon of onion powder
- ¼ teaspoon of cayenne pepper
- ¼ teaspoon of ground turmeric
- Salt and ground black pepper, as required
- 2 (7-ounce of) boneless, skinless chicken breasts, pounded into ¾-inch thickness
- 1 tablespoon of extra-virgin olive oil

For Salad:

- 5 cups of fresh kale, tough ribs removed and chopped
- 1 cup of cucumber, chopped
- ½ cup of red onion, sliced
- ¼ cup of pine nuts

For Dressing:

- 1 small garlic clove, minced
- 2 tablespoons of fresh lemon juice
- 2 tablespoons of extra-virgin olive oil
- 1 teaspoon of maple syrup
- Salt and ground black pepper, as required

Instructions:

1. Preheat your oven to 425 degrees F. Line a baking dish with parchment paper.
2. For chicken: In a bowl, mix together the thyme, spices, salt, and black pepper.
3. Drizzle the chicken breasts with oil, then rub with spice mixture generously and drizzle with the oil.
4. Arrange the chicken breasts onto the prepared baking dish.
5. Bake for about 16-18 minutes.
6. Remove pan from oven and place the chicken breasts onto a chopping board for about 5 minutes.
7. For Salad: Place all ingredients in a salad bowl and blend.
8. For Dressing: Place all ingredients in another bowl and beat until well combined.
9. Cut each chicken breast into desired sized slices.
10. Place the Salad onto each serving plate and top each with chicken slices.
11. Drizzle with dressing and serve.

Turkey & Veggie Salad

Servings: 4

Preparation Time: 15 minutes

Ingredients:

For Salad:

- 3 cups of cooked turkey meat, chopped
- 2 cups of cucumber, chopped
- 1 cup of cherry tomatoes, halved
- 1 cup of radishes, trimmed and sliced
- 6 cups of fresh baby arugula
- 4 tablespoons of scallion greens, chopped
- 4 tablespoons of fresh parsley leaves, chopped

For Dressing:

- 1 garlic clove, minced
- 3 tablespoons of extra-virgin olive oil
- 1 tablespoon of balsamic vinegar
- 1 tablespoon of fresh lemon juice
- Salt and ground black pepper, as required

Instructions:

1. For Salad: In a large serving bowl, add all the ingredients and blend.
2. For Dressing: In another bowl, add all the ingredients and beat till well combined.
3. Pour dressing over Salad and gently toss to coat well.
4. Serve immediately.

Ground Turkey Salad

Servings: 6

Preparation Time: 20minutes

Cooking Time: 13 minutes

Ingredients:

- 1-pound ground turkey
- 1 tablespoon of olive oil
- Salt and ground black pepper, as required
- ¼ cup of water
- ½ of English cucumber, chopped
- 4 cups of green cabbage, shredded
- ½ cup of fresh mint leaves, chopped
- 2 tablespoons of fresh lime juice
- ¼ cup of walnuts, chopped

Instructions:

1. Heat oil in a large skillet over medium-high heat and cook the turkey for about 6-8 minutes, ending the pieces with a spatula.

2. Stir in the water and cook for about 4-5 minutes or until most of the liquid is evaporated.

3. Remove from the heat and transfer the turkey into a bowl.

4. Set the bowl aside to chill completely.

5. In a large serving bowl, add the vegetables, mint, and lime juice and blend well.

6. Add the cooked turkey and stir to mix.

7. Serve immediately.

Steak & Tomato Salad

Servings: 5

Preparation Time: 15 minutes

Cooking Time: 15 minutes

Ingredients:

For Steak:

- 2 tablespoons of fresh oregano, chopped
- ½ tablespoon of garlic, minced
- 1 tablespoon of fresh lemon peel, grated
- ½ teaspoon of red pepper flakes, crushed
- Salt and ground black pepper, as required
- 1 (1-pound) (1-inch thick) boneless beef top sirloin steak

For Salad:

- 6 cups of fresh salad greens
- 2 cups of cherry tomatoes, halved
- 2 tablespoons of olive oil
- 2 tablespoons of fresh lime juice
- Salt and ground black pepper, as required

Instructions:

1. Preheat the gas grill to medium heat.
2. Lightly grease the grill grate.
3. For steak: in a bowl, add the oregano, garlic, lemon rind, red pepper flakes, salt, and black pepper and blend well.
4. Rub the steak with garlic mixture evenly.
5. Place the steak onto the grill and cook, covered for about 12-17 minutes, flipping occasionally.
6. Remove the steak from the grill and place it onto a chopping board for about 10 minutes.
7. Meanwhile, For Salad: In a large serving bowl, place all ingredients and toss to coat well.
8. Cut the steak into bite-sized pieces.
9. Add the steak pieces into the bowl of Salad and toss to coat well.
10. Serve immediately.

Steak, Egg & Veggies Salad

Servings: 4

Preparation Time: 20 minutes

Cooking Time: 9 minutes

Ingredients:

For Steak:

- 2 tablespoons of extra-virgin olive oil
- 1-pound flank steak, sliced thinly
- Salt and ground black pepper, as required

For Salad:

- 4 hard-boiled eggs, peeled and halved
- 1 cup of radishes, cut into matchsticks
- 1 cup of cucumber, cut into matchsticks
- 1 cup of tomato, chopped
- ½ cup of scallion greens, chopped

For Dressing:

- ¼ cup of fresh orange juice
- 3 tablespoons of extra-virgin olive oil
- 2 tablespoons of low-sodium soy sauce

- 2 tablespoons of white vinegar
- 1 tablespoon of fresh lime juice
- 1 tablespoon of maple syrup
- 1 teaspoon of fresh lime zest, grated
- 1 garlic clove, minced

Instructions:

1. Heat oil in a large heavy-bottomed pan over medium-high heat and sear the meat slices with salt and black pepper for about 4-5 minutes or until cooked through.
2. Transfer the meat slices onto a plate and put aside.
3. Meanwhile, in a pan of lightly salted boiling water, cook the noodles for about 5 minutes.
4. Drain the noodles well and rinse under cold water.
5. Drain the noodles again.
6. For Dressing: In a bowl, add all ingredients and beat until well combined.
7. Divide beef slices, noodles, veggies, and scallion into serving bowls and drizzle with dressing.
8. Serve immediately.

Steak & Kale Salad

Servings: 2

Preparation Time: 15 minutes

Cooking Time: 8 minutes

Ingredients:

For Steak:

- 2 teaspoons of olive oil
- 2 (4-ounce of) strip steaks
- Salt and ground black pepper, as required

For Salad:

- ½ cup of carrot, peeled and shredded
- ½ cup of cucumber, peeled, seeded, and sliced
- 3 cups of fresh kale, tough ribs removed and chopped

For Dressing:

- 1 tablespoon of extra-virgin olive oil
- 1 tablespoon of fresh lemon juice
- Salt and ground black pepper, as required

Instructions:

1. For steak: in a large heavy-bottomed skillet, heat the oil over high heat and cook the steaks with salt and black pepper for about 3-4 minutes per side.
2. Transfer the steaks onto a chopping board for about 5 minutes before slicing.
3. For Salad: place all ingredients in a salad bowl and blend.
4. For Dressing: Place all ingredients in another bowl and beat until well combined.
5. Cut the steaks into desired sized slices against the grain.
6. Place the Salad onto each serving plate.
7. Top each plate with steak slices.
8. Drizzle with dressing and serve.

Steak & Veggie Salad

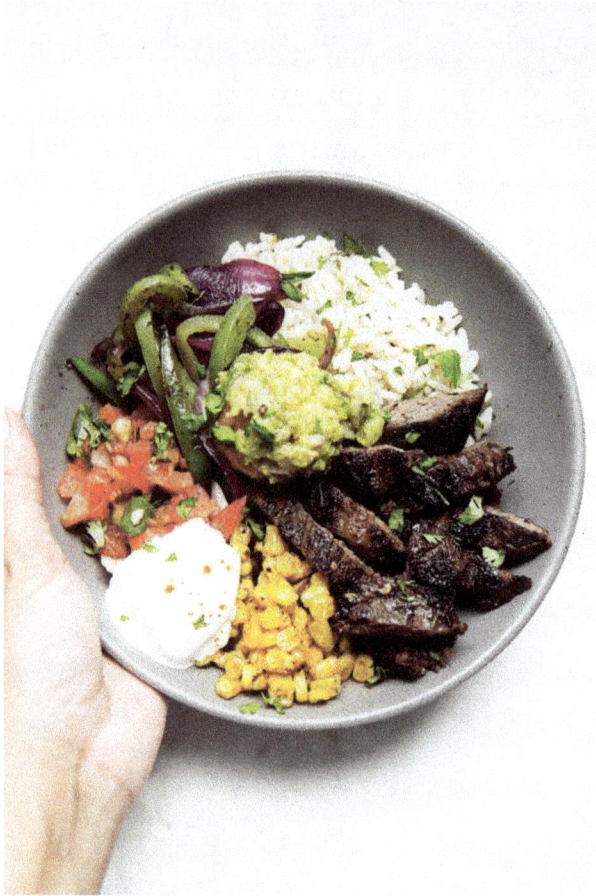

Servings: 8

Preparation Time: 20 minutes

Cooking Time: 16 minutes

Ingredients:

For Steak:

- 2 garlic cloves, crushed
- 1 teaspoon of fresh ginger, grated
- 1 tablespoon of honey
- 2 tablespoons of olive oil
- Salt and freshly ground black pepper, to taste
- 1½ pounds of flank steak, trimmed

For Dressing:

- 1 garlic clove, minced
- 4 tablespoons of extra-virgin olive oil
- 3 tablespoons of fresh lime juice
- ¼ teaspoon of red pepper flakes, crushed
- Salt and freshly ground black pepper, to taste

For Salad:

- 3 cup of cucumber, sliced
- 3 cup of cherry tomatoes, halved
- 1 cup of red onion, sliced thinly
- 4 tablespoons of fresh mint leaves
- 8 cup of fresh spinach, torn

Instructions:

1. For steak: in a large sealable bag, mix all ingredients except steak.

2. Add steak and coat with marinade generously.

3. Seal the bag and refrigerate to marinate for about 24 hours.

4. Remove from the refrigerator and put aside in temperature for about 15 minutes.

5. Heat a Lightly greased grill pan over medium-high heat and cook the steak for about 6-8 minutes per side.

6. Remove the steak from the grill pan and place it onto a chopping board for about 10 minutes before slicing.

7. For Dressing: In a small bowl, add all ingredients and beat well.

8. For Salad: In a large salad bowl, mix together all ingredients.

9. With a pointy knife, cut into desired slices.

10. Divide Salad onto serving plates and top with steak slices.

11. Drizzle with dressing and serve immediately.

Salmon & Veggie Salad

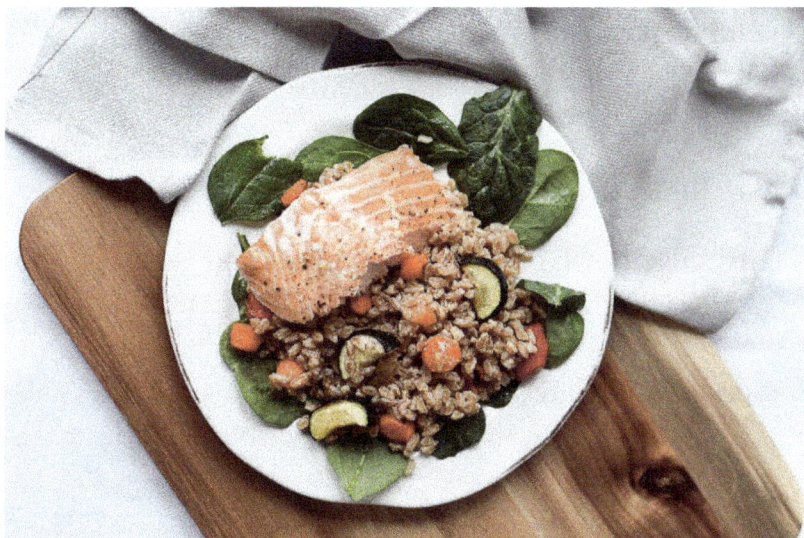

Servings: 2

Preparation Time: 15 minutes

Ingredients:

- 6 ounces of cooked wild salmon, chopped
- 1 cup of cucumber, sliced
- 1 cup of red bell pepper, seeded and sliced
- ½ cup of grape tomatoes, quartered
- 1 tablespoon of scallion green, chopped
- 1 cup of lettuce, torn

- 1 cup of fresh spinach, torn
- 2 tablespoons of olive oil
- 2 tablespoons of fresh lemon juice

Instructions:

1. In a salad bowl, place all ingredients and gently toss to coat well.

2. Serve immediately.

Tuna Salad

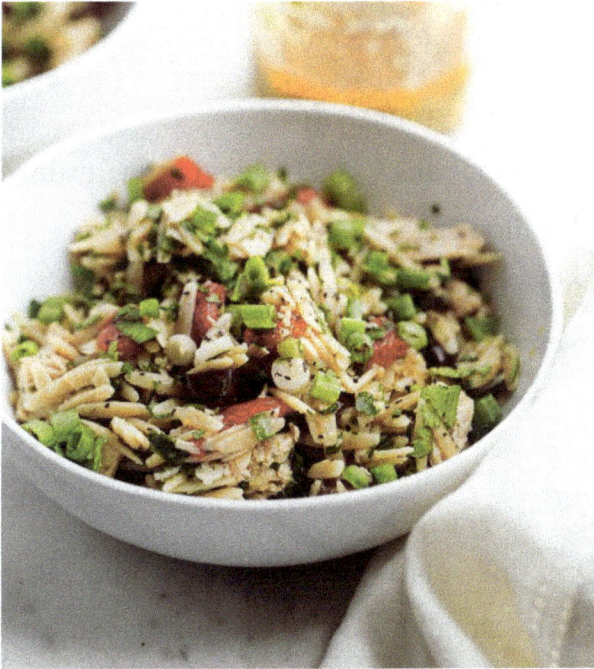

Servings: 4

Preparation Time: 15 minutes

Ingredients:

For Dressing:

- 2 tablespoons of fresh dill, minced
- 2 tablespoons of olive oil

- 1 tablespoon of fresh lime juice
- Salt and ground black pepper, to taste

For Salad:

- 4 cups of fresh spinach, torn
- 2 (6-ounce of) cans water-packed tuna, drained and flaked
- 6 hard-boiled eggs, peeled and sliced
- 1 cup of tomato, chopped
- 1 large cucumber, sliced

Instructions:

1. For Dressing: place dill, oil, lemon juice, salt, and black pepper in a small bowl and beat until well combined.
2. Divide the spinach onto serving plates and top each with tuna, egg, cucumber, and tomato.
3. Drizzle with dressing and serve.

Shrimp & Greens Salad

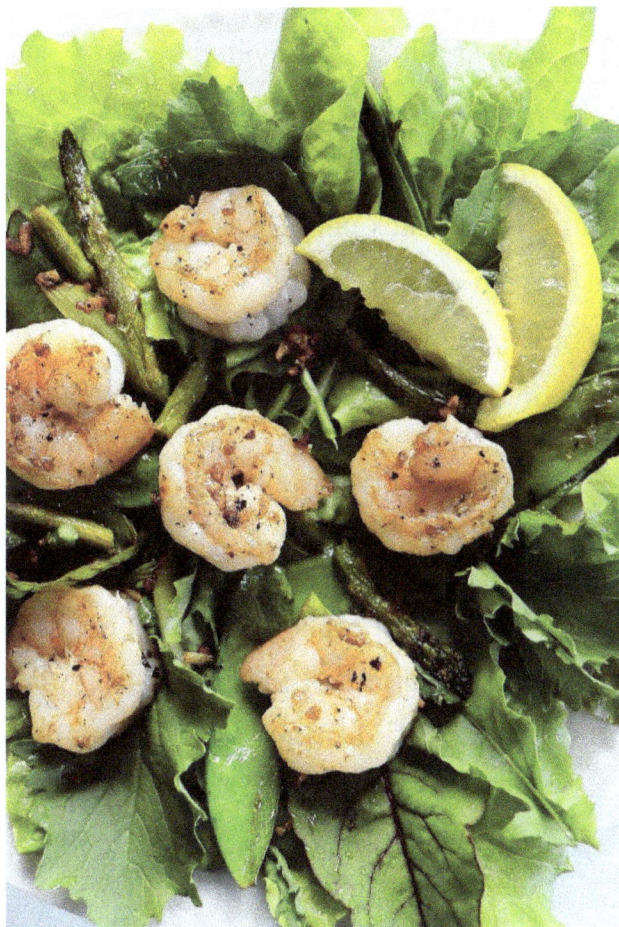

Servings: 6

Preparation Time: 15 minutes

Cooking Time: 6 minutes

Ingredients:

- 3 tablespoons of olive oil, divided
- 1 garlic clove, crushed and divided
- 2 tablespoons of fresh rosemary, chopped
- 1-pound shrimp, peeled and deveined
- Salt and ground black pepper, as required
- 4 cups of fresh arugula
- 2 cups of lettuce, torn
- 2 tablespoons of fresh lime juice

Instructions:

1. In a large wok, heat 1 tablespoon of oil over medium heat and sauté 1 clove for about 1 minute.
2. Add the shrimp with salt and black pepper and cook for about 4-5 minutes.
3. Remove from the heat and put aside to chill.
4. Ina large bowl, add the shrimp, arugula, remaining oil, lime juice, salt, and black pepper, and gently toss to coat.
5. Serve immediately.

Shrimp, Apple & Carrot Salad

Servings: 4

Preparation Time: 20 minutes

Cooking Time: 3 minutes

Ingredients:

- 12 medium shrimp
- 1½ cups of Granny Smith apple, cored and sliced thinly
- 1½ cups of carrot, peeled and cut into matchsticks
- ½ cup of fresh mint leaves, chopped
- 2 tablespoons of balsamic vinegar
- ¼ cup of extra-virgin olive oil
- 1 teaspoon of lemongrass, chopped
- 1 teaspoon of garlic, minced
- 2 sprigs fresh cilantro, leaves separated and chopped

Instructions:

1. In a large pan of salted boiling water, add the shrimp and lemon and cook for about 3 minutes.
2. Remove from the heat and drain the shrimp well.
3. Put aside to chill.

4. After cooling, peel and devein the shrimps.

5. Transfer the shrimp into a large bowl.

6. Add the remaining all ingredients except cilantro and gently stir to mix.

7. Cover the bowl and refrigerate for about 1 hour.

8. Top with cilantro just before serving.

Shrimp & Green Beans Salad

Servings: 5

Preparation Time: 20 minutes

Cooking Time: 8 minutes

Ingredients:

For Shrimp:

- 2 tablespoons of olive oil
- 2 tablespoons of fresh key lime juice
- 4 large garlic cloves, peeled
- 2 sprigs of fresh rosemary leaves
- ½ teaspoon of garlic salt
- 20 large shrimp, peeled and deveined

For Salad:

- 1-pound fresh green beans, trimmed
- ¼ cup of olive oil
- 1 onion, sliced
- Salt and ground black pepper, as required
- ½ cup of garlic and herb feta cheese, crumbled

Instructions:

1. For shrimp marinade: In a blender, add all the ingredients except shrimp and pulse until smooth.
2. Transfer the marinade to a large bowl.
3. Add the shrimp and coat with marinade generously.
4. Cover the bowl and refrigerate to marinate for at least 30 minutes.
5. Preheat the broiler in the oven. Arrange the rack in the top position of the oven. Line a large baking sheet with a bit of foil.
6. Place the shrimp with marinade onto the prepared baking sheet.
7. Broil for about 3-4 minutes per side.
8. Transfer the shrimp mixture into a bowl and refrigerate until using.
9. Meanwhile, For Salad: in a pan of the salted boiling water, add the green beans and cook for about 3-4 minutes.
10. Drain the green beans well and rinse under cold running water.
11. Transfer the green beans into a large bowl.
12. Add the onion, shrimp, salt, and black pepper and stir to mix.
13. Cover and refrigerate to relax for about 1 hour.
14. Stir in cheese just before serving.

Shrimp & Olives Salad

Servings: 4

Preparation Time: 15 minutes

Cooking Time: 3 minutes

Ingredients:

- 1-pound shrimp, peeled and deveined
- 1 lemon, quartered
- 2 tablespoons of olive oil
- 2 teaspoons of fresh lemon juice
- Salt and freshly ground black pepper, to taste
- 2 tomatoes, sliced
- ¼ cup of onion, sliced
- ¼ cup of green olives
- ¼ cup of fresh cilantro, chopped finely

Instructions:

1. In a pan of lightly salted boiling water, add the quartered lemon.
2. Then, add the shrimp and cook for about 2-3 minutes or until pink and opaque.

3. With a slotted spoon, transfer the shrimp into a bowl of drinking water to prevent the cooking process.
4. Drain the shrimp completely, then pat dry with paper towels.
5. In a small bowl, add the oil, lemon juice, salt, and black pepper, and beat until well combined.
6. Divide the shrimp, tomato, onion, olives, and cilantro onto serving plates.
7. Drizzle with oil mixture and serve.

Shrimp & Arugula Salad

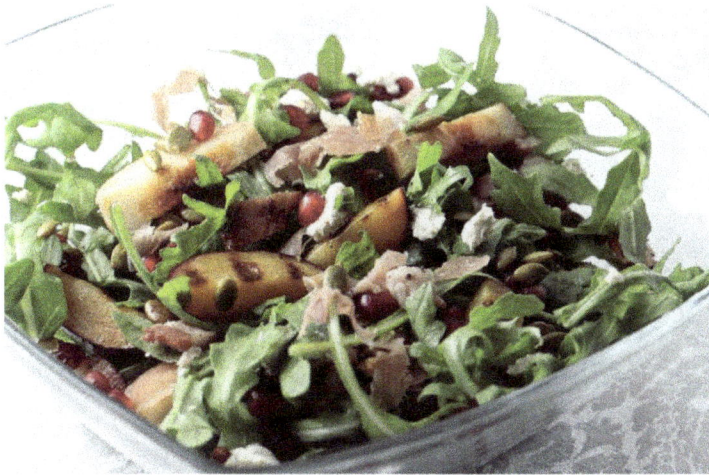

Servings: 4

Preparation Time: 15 minutes

Cooking Time: 5 minutes

Ingredients:

For Shrimp:

- 1-pound large shrimp, peeled and deveined
- ½ tablespoon of fresh lemon juice

For Salad:

- 6 cups of fresh arugula

- 2 tablespoons of extra-virgin olive oil
- 1 tablespoon of fresh lemon juice
- Salt and ground black pepper, as required

Instructions:

1. In a large pan of salted boiling water, add the shrimp and juice and cook for about 2 minutes.
2. With a slotted spoon, remove the shrimp from the pan and place it into an ice bath.
3. Drain the shrimp well.
4. In a large bowl, add the shrimp, arugula, oil, juice, salt, black pepper, and gently toss to coat.
5. Serve immediately.

Shrimp & Veggies Salad

Servings: 6

Preparation Time: 20 minutes

Cooking Time: 5 minutes

Ingredients:

For Dressing:

- 2 tablespoons of natural almond butter
- 1 garlic clove, crushed
- 1 tablespoon of fresh cilantro, chopped
- 2 tablespoons of fresh lime juice
- 1 tablespoon of maple syrup
- ½ teaspoon of cayenne pepper
- ¼ teaspoon of salt
- 1 tablespoon of water
- 1/3 cup of olive oil

For Salad:

- 1-pound shrimp, peeled and deveined
- Salt and ground black pepper, as required
- 1 teaspoon of olive oil

- 1 cup of carrot, peeled and julienned
- 1 cup of red cabbage, shredded
- 1 cup of green cabbage, shredded
- 1 cup of cucumber, julienned
- 4 cups of fresh baby arugula
- ¼ cup of fresh basil, chopped
- ¼ cup of fresh cilantro, chopped
- 4 cups of lettuce, torn
- ¼ cup of almonds, chopped

Instructions:

1. For Dressing: In a bowl, add all ingredients except oil and beat until well combined.
2. Slowly add oil, beating continuously until smooth.
3. For Salad: In a bowl, add shrimp, salt, black pepper, and oil and toss to coat well.
4. Heat a skillet over medium-high heat and cook shrimp for about 2 minutes per side.
5. Remove from the heat and put aside to chill.
6. In a large serving bowl, add all the cooked shrimp, remaining salad ingredients, and dressing and toss to coat well.
7. Serve immediately.

Scallop & Tomato Salad

Servings: 4

Preparation Time: 15 minutes

Cooking Time: 6 minutes

Ingredients:

For Scallops:

- 1¼ pounds fresh sea scallops, side muscles removed
- Salt and freshly ground black pepper, to taste
- 2 tablespoons of olive oil
- 1 garlic clove, minced

For Salad

- 6 cup of mixed baby greens
- ¼ cup of yellow grape tomatoes halved
- ¼ cup of red grape tomatoes halved
- 2 tablespoons of olive oil
- 2 tablespoons of fresh lemon juice
- Salt and freshly ground black pepper, to taste

Instructions:

1. Sprinkle the scallops with salt and black pepper evenly.
2. In a large skillet, heat the oil over medium-high heat and cook the scallops for about 2-3 minutes per side.
3. Meanwhile, For Salad: In a bowl, add all ingredients and toss to coat well.
4. Divide the salad onto serving plates.
5. Top each plate with scallops and serve.

Tofu & Veggie Salad

Servings: 8

Preparation Time: 20 minutes

Ingredients:

For Dressing:

- ¼ cup of balsamic vinegar
- ¼ cup of low-sodium soy sauce
- 2 tablespoons of water
- 1 teaspoon of sesame oil, toasted
- 1 teaspoon of Sriracha
- 3-4 drops of liquid stevia

For Salad:

1. 1½ pounds baked firm tofu, cubed
2. 2 large zucchinis, sliced thinly
3. 2 large yellow bell peppers, seeded and sliced thinly
4. 3 cups of cherry tomatoes, halved
5. 2 cups of radishes, sliced thinly
6. 2 cups of purple cabbage, shredded
7. 10 cups of fresh baby spinach

Instructions:

1. For Dressing: In a bowl, add all the ingredients and beat until well combined.

2. Divide the chickpeas, tofu, and vegetables into serving bowls.

3. Drizzle with dressing and serve immediately.

Chicken & Kale Soup

Servings: 4

Preparation Time: 15 minutes

Cooking Time: 15 minutes

Ingredients:

- 2 tablespoons of extra-virgin olive oil
- ½ of medium onion, chopped
- 3 garlic cloves, minced
- 4 cups of homemade low-sodium chicken broth
- 1 cup of cooked chicken, cubed
- 1 bunch fresh kale, tough ribs removed and chopped
- 2 tablespoons of fresh lemon juice
- Salt and ground black pepper, to taste

Instructions:

1. In a soup pan, heat vegetable oil over medium-high heat and sauté the onion and garlic for about 2-3 minutes.
2. Stir in the cooked chicken and broth and bring to a mild boil.

3. Now, adjust the heat and to low and simmer for about 3 minutes.

4. Stir in the kale and simmer for five minutes or until the kale is tender.

5. Stir in the lemon juice, salt, and black pepper and take away from the heat.

6. Serve hot.

Chicken & Spinach Stew

Servings: 8

Preparation Time: 15 minutes

Cooking Time: 30 minutes

Ingredients:

- 2 tablespoons of olive oil
- 1 yellow onion, chopped
- 1 tablespoon of garlic, minced
- 1 tablespoon of fresh ginger, minced
- 1 teaspoon of ground turmeric
- 1 teaspoon of ground cumin
- 1 teaspoon of ground coriander
- 1 teaspoon of paprika
- 1 teaspoon of cayenne pepper
- 6 (4-ounce of) boneless, skinless chicken thighs, trimmed and cut into 1-inch pieces
- 4 tomatoes, chopped
- 1 (14-ounce of) can unsweetened coconut milk
- Salt and ground black pepper, to taste
- 3 cups of fresh spinach, chopped

Instructions:

1. In a large heavy-bottomed pan, heat the oil over medium heat and sauté the onion for about 3-4 minutes.

2. Add the ginger, garlic, and spices, and sauté for about 1 minute.

3. Add the chicken and cook for about 4-5 minutes.

4. Add the tomatoes, coconut milk, salt, and black pepper and bring it to a gentle simmer.

5. Now, adjust the heat to low and simmer, covered for about 10-15 minutes.

6. Stir in the spinach and cook for about 4–5 minutes.

7. Remove from the heat and serve hot.

Turkey Meatballs & Kale Soup

Servings: 6

Preparation Time: 20 minutes

Cooking Time: 25 minutes

Ingredients:

For Meatballs:

- 1-pound lean ground turkey
- 1 garlic clove, minced
- 1 egg, beaten
- ¼ cup of low-fat Parmesan cheese, grated
- Salt and ground black pepper, as required

For Soup:

- 1 tablespoon of olive oil
- 1 small yellow onion, chopped finely
- 1 garlic clove, minced
- 6 cups of low-sodium chicken broth
- 8 cups of fresh kale, trimmed and chopped
- 2 eggs, beaten lightly
- Salt and ground black pepper, as required

Instructions:

1. For meatballs: in a bowl, add all ingredients and blend until well combined.
2. Make equal-sized small balls from the mixture.
3. In a large soup pan, heat oil over medium heat and sauté onion for about 5-6 minutes.
4. Add the garlic and sauté for about 1 minute.
5. Add the broth and bring to a boil.
6. Carefully place the balls in the pan and bring to a boil.
7. Reduce the heat to low and cook for about 10 minutes.
8. Stir in the kale and bring the soup to a mild simmer.
9. Simmer for about 2-3 minutes.
10. Slowly add the beaten eggs, stirring continuously.
11. Cook for about 1-2 minutes, stirring continuously.
12. Season with salt and black pepper and take away from the heat.

13. Serve hot.

Turkey & Spinach Stew

Servings: 4

Preparation Time: 15 minutes

Cooking Time: 35 minutes

Ingredients:

- 2 tablespoons of extra-virgin olive oil
- 1 medium onion, chopped
- 2 cups of carrots, peeled and chopped
- 2 large tomatoes, peeled, seeded, and chopped final
- 1 teaspoon of ground cumin
- ½ teaspoon of red pepper flakes, crushed
- 2 cups of low-sodium vegetable broth
- 2 cups of cooked turkey meat, chopped
- 3 cups of fresh spinach, chopped
- 1 tablespoon of fresh lemon juice
- Salt and ground black pepper, to taste

Instructions:

1. Heat vegetable oil in a large soup pan over medium heat and sauté the onion and carrot for about 6-8 minutes.
2. Add the tomatoes, cumin, and red pepper flakes and cook for about 2-3 minutes.
3. Add the broth and bring to a boil.
4. Adjust the heat to low and simmer for about 10 minutes.
5. Stir in the chickpeas and simmer for about 5 minutes.
6. Stir in the kale and simmer for 4-5 minutes more.
7. Stir in the lemon juice, salt, and black pepper and take away from the heat.

8. Serve hot.

Turkey & Mushroom Stew

Servings: 10

Preparation Time: 15 minutes

Cooking Time: 3 hours 10 minutes

Ingredients:

- 2 pounds turkey thigh and leg meat, chopped
- 2 tablespoons of olive oil
- 1 garlic clove, crushed
- 12 ounces of fresh button mushrooms
- 2 scallions, sliced
- 2 tablespoons of fresh thyme leaves
- Salt and ground white pepper, as required
- 1 cup of full-fat coconut milk
- 2 tablespoons of whole grain mustard
- 1 teaspoon of xanthan gum
- ½ cup of fresh parsley, roughly chopped

Instructions:

1. Heat a non-stick skillet over high heat and cook the turkey meat for about 4-5 minutes or until browned completely.
2. Transfer the turkey meat into a slow cooker.
3. In the same skillet, heat the oil and sauté the mushrooms and scallion for about 3-5 minutes.
4. Transfer the mushroom mixture into the slow cooker alongside the thyme, salt, and black pepper.
5. In a bowl, add the coconut milk, mustard, and xanthan gum and beat until well combined.
6. Add the coconut milk mixture into the slow cooker and stir to mix well.
7. Set the slow cooker on High and cook, covered for about 3 hours.
8. Uncover and sir in the parsley.
9. Serve hot.

Beef & Bok Choy Soup

Servings: 6

Preparation Time: 15 minutes

Cooking Time: 30 minutes

Ingredients:

- 1 tablespoon of olive oil
- 1-pound of ground beef
- ½ pound of fresh mushrooms, sliced
- 1 small yellow onion, chopped
- 1 garlic clove, minced
- 1-pound head bok choy, stalks and leaves separated and chopped
- 2 tablespoons of low-sodium soy sauce
- 5 cups of low-sodium chicken broth
- Freshly ground black pepper, to taste

Instructions:

1. In a large pan, heat oil over medium-high heat and cook the meat for about 5 minutes.

2. Add the onion, mushrooms, garlic and cook for about 5 minutes.

3. Add the bok choy stalks and cook for about 4-5 minutes.

4. Add soy and broth and bring to a boil.

5. Reduce the heat to low. Cover and cook for about 10 minutes.

6. Stir in the bok choy leaves and cook for about 5 minutes.

7. Stir in black pepper and serve hot.

Beef & Cabbage Stew

Servings: 8

Preparation Time: 15 minutes

Cooking Time: 1 hour 50 minutes

Ingredients:

- 2 pounds beef stew meat, trimmed and cubed into 1-inch size
- 1 1/3 cups of homemade hot low-sodium chicken broth
- 2 yellow onions, chopped
- 2 bay leaves
- 1 teaspoon of Greek seasoning
- Salt and ground black pepper, as required
- 3 celery stalks, chopped
- 1 (8-ounce of) package shredded cabbage
- 1 (6-ounce of) can sugar-free tomato sauce
- 1 (8-ounce of) can sugar-free whole plum tomatoes, chopped roughly with liquid

Instructions:

1. Heat a large nonstick pan over medium-high heat and cook the meat for about 4-5 minutes or until browned.

2. Drain excess grease from the pan.

3. Stir in the broth, onion, bay leaves, Greek seasoning, salt, and black pepper, and bring to a boil.

4. Reduce the heat to low and cook, covered for about 1¼ hours.

5. Stir in the celery and cabbage and cook, covered for about 30 minutes.

6. Stir in the spaghetti sauce and chopped plum tomatoes and cook, uncovered for about 15-20 minutes.

7. Stir in the salt and take away from heat.

8. Discard bay leaves and serve hot.

Beef & Carrot Stew

Servings: 6

Preparation Time: 15 minutes

Cooking Time: 55 minutes

Ingredients:

- 1½ pounds beef stew meat, trimmed and chopped
- Salt and ground black pepper, to taste
- 1 tablespoon of olive oil
- 1 cup of homemade tomato puree
- 4 cups of homemade low-sodium beef broth
- 3 carrots, peeled and sliced
- 2 garlic cloves, minced
- ½ tablespoons of dried thyme
- 1 teaspoon of dried parsley
- 1 teaspoon of dried rosemary
- 1 tablespoon of paprika
- 1 teaspoon of onion powder
- 1 teaspoon of garlic powder
- 3 tablespoons of fresh parsley, chopped

Instructions:

1. In a large bowl, add the meat cubes, salt, and black pepper, and toss to coat well.
2. In a Dutch oven, heat oil over medium-high heat and cook the meat cubes for about 4–5 minutes or until brown.
3. Add in remaining ingredients and stir to mix.
4. Adjust the heat to high and bring to a boil.
5. Now, adjust the heat to low and simmer, covered for about 40–50 minutes.
6. Stir in the salt and black pepper and take away from the heat.
7. Serve hot.

Baked Beef Stew

Servings: 8

Preparation Time: 15 minutes

Cooking Time: 2¼ hours

Ingredients:

- 1 teaspoon of ground coriander
- ¾ teaspoon of ground cumin
- ½ teaspoon of cayenne pepper
- 2 tablespoons of coconut oil
- 3 pounds of beef stew meat, cubed
- Salt and ground black pepper, as required
- ½ yellow onion, chopped
- 2 garlic cloves, minced
- 2 cups of low-sodium chicken broth
- 1 (15-ounce of) can sugar-free diced tomatoes
- 1 medium head cauliflower, cut into 1-inch florets

Instructions:

1. Preheat your oven to 300 degrees F.

2. In a small bowl, mix spices. Set aside.

3. in a large ovenproof pan, heat the oil over medium heat and cook beef with salt and black pepper for about 10 minutes or until browned from all sides.

4. Transfer the meat into a bowl.

5. In the same pan, add the onion and sauté for about 3-4 minutes.

6. Add the garlic and spice mixture and sauté for about 1 minute.

7. Add the cooked beef, broth, and tomatoes and bring to a mild boil.

8. Immediately cover the pan and transfer it into the oven.

9. Bake for about 1½ hours.

10. Remove from the oven and stir in the cauliflower.

11. Bake, covered for about 30 minutes more or until cauliflower is completed completely.

12. Serve hot.

Fish Stew

Servings: 10

Preparation Time: 15 minutes

Cooking Time: 50 minutes

- **Ingredients:**
- ¼ cup of coconut oil
- ½ cup of yellow onion, chopped
- 1 cup of celery stalk, chopped
- ½ cup of green bell pepper, seeded and chopped
- 1 garlic clove, minced
- 4 cups of water
- 4 beef bouillon cubes
- 20 ounces of okra, trimmed and chopped
- 2 (14-ounce of) cans sugar-free diced tomatoes with liquid
- 2 bay leaves
- 1 teaspoon of dried thyme, crushed
- 2 teaspoons of red pepper flakes, crushed
- ¼ teaspoon of hot pepper sauce
- Salt and ground black pepper, as required
- 32 ounces of catfish fillets
- ½ cup of fresh cilantro, chopped

Instructions:

1. In a large skillet, melt the coconut oil over medium heat and sauté the onion, celery, and bell pepper for about 4-5 minutes.

2. Meanwhile, in a large soup pan, mix together bouillon cubes and water and bring to an overboil medium heat.

3. Transfer the onion mixture and remaining ingredients except for catfish into the pan of boiling water and bring to a boil.

4. Reduce the heat to low and cook, covered for about 30 minutes.

5. Stir in catfish fillets and cook for about 10-15 minutes.

6. Stir in the cilantro and take away from the heat.

7. Serve hot.

Shrimp Stew

Servings: 6

Preparation Time: 15 minutes

Cooking Time: 20 minutes

Ingredients:

- ¼ cup of olive oil
- ¼ cup of yellow onion, chopped
- ¼ cup of green bell pepper, seeded and chopped
- 1 garlic clove, minced
- 1½ pounds raw shrimp, peeled and deveined
- 1 (14-ounce of) can diced tomatoes with chilies
- 1 cup of unsweetened coconut milk
- 2 tablespoons of Sriracha
- 2 tablespoons of fresh lime juice
- Salt and ground black pepper, to taste
- ¼ cup of fresh cilantro, chopped

Instructions:

1. Heat oil in a pan over medium heat and sauté the onion for about 4–5 minutes.
2. Add the bell pepper and garlic and sauté for about 4–5 minutes.
3. Add the shrimp and tomatoes and cook for about 3–4 minutes.
4. Stir in the coconut milk and Sriracha and cook for about 4–5 minutes.
5. Stir in the lime juice, salt, and black pepper, and take away from the heat.
6. Garnish with cilantro and serve hot.

Kale & Carrot Soup

Servings: 5

Preparation Time: 15 minutes

Cooking Time: 40 minutes

Ingredients:

- 2 tablespoons of extra-virgin olive oil
- 4 medium carrots, chopped
- 2 celery stalks, chopped
- 1 large red onion, chopped finely
- 2 garlic cloves, crushed
- ½ pound curly kale, tough ribs removed and chopped finely
- 4½ cups of homemade low-sodium vegetable broth
- Salt and ground black pepper, as required

Instructions:

1. Heat the oil in a large soup pan over medium heat and cook the carrot, celery, onion, and garlic for about 8-10 minutes, stirring frequently.
2. Add the kale and cook for about 5 minutes, stirring twice.

3. Add the broth and bring to a boil.

4. Cook, partially covered for about 20 minutes.

5. Stir in salt and black pepper and take away from the heat.

6. With an immersion blender, blend the soup until smooth.

7. Serve hot.

Cheesy Mushroom Soup

Servings: 4

Preparation Time: 15 minutes

Cooking Time: 15 minutes

Ingredients:

- 2 tablespoons of olive oil
- 4 ounces of fresh baby Portobello mushroom, sliced
- 4 ounces of fresh white button mushrooms, sliced
- ½ cup of yellow onion, chopped
- ½ teaspoon of salt
- 1 teaspoon of garlic, chopped
- 3 cups of low-sodium vegetable broth
- 1 cup of low-fat cheddar cheese

Instructions:

1. In a medium pan, heat the oil over medium heat and cook the mushrooms and onion with salt for about 5-7 minutes, stirring frequently.
2. Add the garlic, and sauté for about 1-2 minutes.
3. Stir in the broth and take away from the heat.

4. With a stick blender, blend the soup until mushrooms are chopped very finely.

5. In the pan, add the cream and stir to mix.

6. Place the pan over medium heat and cook for about 3-5 minutes.

7. Remove from the heat and serve immediately.

Spinach & Mushroom Stew

Servings: 4

Preparation Time: 15 minutes

Cooking Time: 30 minutes

Ingredients:

- 2 tablespoons of olive oil
- 2 onions, chopped
- 3 garlic cloves, minced
- ½ pound of fresh button mushrooms, chopped
- ¼ pound of fresh shiitake mushrooms, chopped
- ¼ pound of fresh spinach, chopped
- Sea salt and freshly ground black pepper, to taste
- ¼ cup of low-sodium vegetable broth
- ½ cup of coconut milk
- 2 tablespoons of fresh parsley, chopped

Instructions:

1. In a large skillet, heat oil over medium heat and sauté the onion and garlic for 4-5 minutes.

2. Add the mushrooms, salt, and black pepper and cook for 4-5 minutes.

3. Add the spinach, broth, and coconut milk and bring to a mild boil.

4. Simmer for 4-5 minutes or until desired doneness.

5. Stir in the cilantro and take away from heat.

6. Serve hot.

Veggie Stew

Servings: 4

Preparation Time: 20 minutes

Cooking Time: 35 minutes

Ingredients:

- 2 tablespoons of olive oil
- 1 yellow onion, chopped
- 2 teaspoons of fresh ginger, grated
- 1 teaspoon of ground turmeric
- 1 teaspoon of ground cumin
- Salt and ground black pepper, as required
- 1-2 cups of water, divided
- 1 cup of cabbage, shredded
- 1 cup of broccoli, chopped
- 2 large carrots, peeled and sliced

Instructions:

1. In a large soup pan, heat the oil over medium heat and sauté onion for about 5 minutes.
2. Stir in the ginger and spices and sauté for about 1 minute.

3. Add 1 cup of water and bring to a boil.

4. Reduce the heat to medium-low and cook for about 10 minutes.

5. Add the vegetables and enough water that covers the half vegetable mixture and stir to mix.

6. Increase the heat to medium-high and bring to a boil.

7. Reduce the heat to medium-low and cook, covered for about 10-15 minutes, stirring occasionally.

8. Serve hot.

Tofu & Mushroom Soup

Servings: 3

Preparation Time: 15 minutes

Cooking Time: 25 minutes

Ingredients:

- 3 tablespoons of vegetable oil, divided
- 1 shallot, minced
- 1 ounce of fresh ginger, minced
- 2 garlic cloves, minced
- 5½ ounces of coconut milk
- 1 Roma tomato, chopped
- 1 lemongrass stalk, halved crosswise
- 6 ounces of fresh mushrooms, sliced
- 14 ounces of extra-firm tofu, pressed, drained, and cut into ½-inch cubes
- Ground black pepper, as required
- 1 scallion, sliced
- 1 tablespoon of fresh cilantro

Instructions:

1. In a pan, heat 2 tablespoons of oil over medium-high heat and sauté the shallot, ginger, garlic, and a pinch of salt for about 1-2 minutes.

2. Add coconut milk and remaining water and bring to a boil.

3. Add the tomato and lemongrass and stir to mix.

4. Adjust the heat to low and simmer for about 8-10 minutes.

5. Meanwhile, in a large non-stick skillet, heat the remaining oil over medium-high heat and cook the mushrooms, tofu, pinch of salt, and black pepper for about 5-8 minutes, stirring occasionally.

6. Remove the lemongrass stalk from the pan of soup and discard it.

7. Divide the cooked mushrooms and tofu into serving bowls evenly.

8. Top with hot soup and serve with the garnishing of cilantro.

Tofu & Bell Pepper Stew

Servings: 6

Preparation Time: 15 minutes

Cooking Time: 15 minutes

Ingredients:

- 2 tablespoons of garlic
- 1 jalapeño pepper, seeded and chopped
- 1 (16-ounce of) jar roasted red peppers, rinsed, drained, and chopped
- 2 cups of homemade low-sodium vegetable broth
- 2 cups of filtered water
- 1 medium green bell pepper, seeded and sliced thinly
- 1 medium red bell pepper, seeded and sliced thinly
- 1 (16-ounce of) package extra-firm tofu, drained and cubed
- 1 (10-ounce of) package frozen baby spinach, thawed

Instructions:

1. Add the garlic, jalapeno, and roasted red peppers in a food processor and pulse until smooth.

2. In a large pan, add the puree, broth, and water over medium-high heat and cook until boiling.

3. Add the bell peppers and tofu and stir to mix.

4. Reduce the heat to medium and cook for about 5 minutes.

5. Stir in the spinach and cook for about 5 minutes.

6. Serve hot.

Carrot Soup with Tempeh

Servings: 6

Preparation Time: 15 minutes

Cooking Time: 45 minutes

Ingredients:

- ¼ cup of olive oil, divided
- 1 large yellow onion, chopped
- Salt, as required
- 2 pounds carrots, peeled and cut into ½-inch rounds
- 2 tablespoons of fresh dill, chopped
- 4½ cups of low-sodium vegetable broth
- 12 ounces of tempeh, cut into ½-inch cubes
- ¼ cup of tomato paste
- 1 teaspoon of fresh lemon juice

Instructions:

1. In a large soup pan, heat 2 tablespoons of the oil over medium heat and cook the onion with salt for about 6-8 minutes, stirring frequently.
2. Add the carrots and stir to mix.

3. Lower the heat to low and cook, covered for about 5 minutes, stirring frequently.
4. Add in the broth and bring to an overboil high heat.
5. Lower the heat to a low and simmer, covered for about 30 minutes.
6. Meanwhile, in a skillet, heat the remaining oil over medium-high heat and cook the tempeh for about 35 minutes.
7. Stir in the dill and cook for about 1 minute.
8. Remove from the heat.
9. Remove the pan of soup from heat and stir in tomato paste and lemon juice.
10. With an immersion blender, blend the soup until smooth and creamy.

11. Serve the soup hot with the topping of tempeh.

Chicken Stuffed Avocado

Servings: 2

Preparation Time: 15 minutes

Ingredients:

- 1 cup of cooked chicken, shredded
- 1 avocado, halved and pitted
- 1 tablespoon of fresh lime juice
- ¼ cup of yellow onion, chopped finely
- ¼ cup of low-fat plain Greek yogurt
- Pinch of cayenne pepper
- Salt and ground black pepper, as required

Instructions:

1. With a little scooper, scoop out the flesh from the center of every avocado half and transfer it into a bowl.
2. In the avocado flesh bowl, add the juice, and with a fork, mash until well blended.
3. Add remaining ingredients and stir to mix.
4. Divide the chicken mixture into avocado halves evenly and serve immediately.

Chicken Lettuce Wraps

Servings: 6

Preparation Time: 15 minutes

Cooking Time: 35 minutes

Ingredients:

- 1-pound chicken thighs
- 1 tablespoon of olive oil
- ¼ teaspoon of garlic powder
- Salt and ground black pepper, as required
- 10 romaine lettuce leaves
- ¾ cup of carrot, peeled and julienned
- ¾ cup of cucumber, julienned
- ¼ cup of scallion (green part), chopped

Instructions:

1. Preheat your oven to 390 degrees F. Line a baking sheet with parchment paper.
2. In a bowl, add the chicken, oil, garlic powder, salt, and black pepper and blend well.

3. Arrange the chicken thigh onto the prepared baking sheet in a single layer.

4. Bake for about 20-30 minutes or until desired doneness.

5. Remove from the oven and put aside to chill for about 20 minutes.

6. Cut the cooled chicken thighs into bite-sized pieces.

7. In a bowl, add the chicken pieces, celery, parsley, mayonnaise, salt, and black pepper, and blend until well combined.

8. Arrange the lettuce leaves onto serving plates.

9. Place about ¼ cup of chicken mixture over each lettuce leaf evenly.

10. Top with carrot, cucumber, and scallion and serve.

Chicken & Strawberry Lettuce Wraps

Servings: 2

Preparation Time: 15 minutes

Ingredients:

- 6 ounces of cooked chicken breast, cut into strips
- ½ cup of fresh strawberries, hulled and sliced thinly
- 1 English cucumber, sliced thinly
- 1 tablespoon of fresh mint leaves, minced
- 4 large lettuce leaves

Instructions

1. In a large bowl, add all ingredients except lettuce leaves and gently toss to coat well.
2. Place the lettuce leaves onto serving plates.
3. Place the chicken mixture over each lettuce leaf evenly and serve immediately.

Ground Chicken Lettuce Wraps

Servings: 5

Preparation Time: 15 minutes

Cooking Time: 15 minutes

Ingredients:

<u>For Chicken:</u>

- 2 tablespoons of avocado oil
- 1 small onion, chopped finely
- 1 teaspoon of fresh ginger, minced
- 2 garlic cloves, minced
- 1¼ pounds of ground chicken
- Salt and ground black pepper, to taste

<u>For Wraps:</u>

- 10 romaine lettuce leaves
- 1½ cups of carrot, peeled and julienned
- 2 tablespoons of fresh parsley, chopped finely
- 2 tablespoons of fresh lime juice

Instructions:

1. In a skillet, heat the oil over medium heat and sauté the onion, ginger, and garlic for about 4-5 minutes.
2. Add the ground chicken, salt, and black pepper, and cook over medium-high heat for about 7-9 minutes, ending the meat into smaller pieces with a wooden spoon.
3. Remove from the heat and put aside to chill.
4. Arrange the lettuce leaves onto serving plates.
5. Place the cooked chicken over each lettuce leaf and top with carrot and cilantro.
6. Drizzle with juice and serve immediately.

Chicken Burgers

Servings: 4

Preparation Time: 15 minutes

Cooking Time: 10 minutes

Ingredients:

For Burgers:

- 1¼ pounds ground chicken
- 1 egg
- ½ yellow onion, grated
- Salt and ground black pepper, as required
- 1 teaspoon of dried thyme
- 2 tablespoons of olive oil

For Serving:

- 4 cups of lettuce, torn
- 1 cucumber, chopped

Instructions:

1. In a bowl, add all the ingredients and blend until well combined.
2. Make 8 small equal-sized patties from the mixture.
3. In a large frying pan, heat the oil over medium heat and cook the patties for about 4-5 minutes per side or until done completely.
4. Divide the lettuce and cucumber onto serving plates and top each with 2 burgers.
5. Serve hot.

Chicken & Avocado Burgers

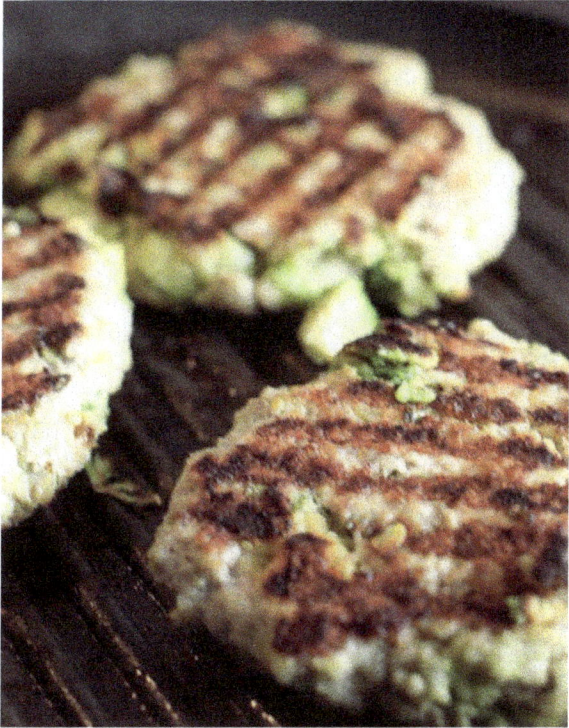

Servings: 4

Preparation Time: 15 minutes

Cooking Time: 10 minutes

Ingredients:

- ½ of ripe avocado, peeled, pitted, and cut into chunks

- ½ cup of low-fat Parmesan cheese, grated
- 1 garlic clove, minced
- Freshly ground black pepper, to taste
- 1-pound lean ground chicken
- Olive oil cooking spray
- 6 cups of fresh baby green

Instructions:

1. In a bowl, add the avocado chunks, Parmesan cheese, garlic, and black pepper, and toss to coat well.
2. Add the ground chicken and gently stir to mix.
3. Make 4 equal-sized patties from the chicken mixture.
4. Heat a greased grill pan over medium heat.
5. Place the patties into the grill pan and cook for about 5 minutes per side.
6. Divide the greens onto serving plates and top each with 1 burger.
7. Serve immediately.

Chicken Meatballs with Mash

Servings: 4

Preparation Time: 20 minutes

Cooking Time: 10 minutes

Ingredients:

For Meatballs:

- 1-pound ground chicken
- 2 garlic cloves, minced
- 1 large egg, beaten
- ½ cup of low-fat Parmesan cheese, grated freshly
- 2 tablespoons of fresh parsley, chopped
- Salt and ground black pepper, as required
- 2 tablespoons of olive oil

For Broccoli Mash:

- 1½ cups of broccoli florets
- 2 tablespoons of fresh basil, chopped finely
- 1 tablespoon of coconut oil, softened
- 1 garlic clove, minced
- Salt and ground black pepper, as required

- For Serving:
- ¼ cup of black olives
- 1 cup of fresh baby spinach leaves
- ½ of lemon, cut into slices

Instructions:

1. For meatballs: in a large bowl, add all ingredients apart from oil and sesame seeds and with your hands, mix until well combined.
2. Make small equal-sized balls from the mixture.
3. In a non-stick skillet, heat oil over medium heat and cook the meatballs for about 10 minutes or until done completely.
4. With a slotted spoon, transfer the meatballs onto a paper towel-lined plate to drain.
5. Meanwhile, for broccoli mash: in a pan of the lightly salted boiling water, add the broccoli and cook for about 2-3 minutes.
6. Remove from the heat and drain the broccoli completely.
7. In a food processor, add the broccoli and remaining ingredients and pulse until smooth.
8. Divide the broccoli mash onto serving plates and top with meatballs, olives, spinach, and lemon slices.
9. Serve immediately.

Chicken & Veggie Skewers

Servings: 6

Preparation Time: 15 minutes

Cooking Time: 8 minutes

Ingredients:

- ¼ cup of low-fat Parmigiano Reggiano cheese, grated
- 3 tablespoons of olive oil
- 2 garlic cloves, minced
- 1 cup of fresh basil leaves, chopped
- Salt and ground black pepper, to taste
- 1¼ pounds boneless, skinless chicken breast, cut into 1-inch cubes
- 1 large green bell pepper, seeded and cubed
- 24 cherry tomatoes

Instructions:

1. Add cheese, butter, garlic, basil, salt, and black pepper in a food processor and pulse until smooth.
2. Transfer the basil mixture into a large bowl.
3. Add the chicken cubes and blend well.

4. Cover the bowl and refrigerate to marinate for at least 4-5 hours.

5. Preheat the grill to medium-high heat. Generously, grease the grill grate.

6. Thread the chicken, bell pepper cubes, and tomatoes onto presoaked wooden skewers.

7. Place the skewers onto the grill and cook for about 6-8 minutes, flipping occasionally.

8. Remove from the grill and place onto a platter for about 5 minutes before serving.

Stuffed Chicken Breast

Servings: 4

Preparation Time: 15 minutes

Cooking Time: 25 minutes

Ingredients:

- 1 tablespoon of olive oil
- 1 small onion, chopped
- 1 pepperoni pepper, seeded and sliced thinly
- ½ of red bell pepper, seeded and sliced thinly
- 2 teaspoons of garlic, minced
- 1 cup of fresh spinach, trimmed and chopped
- ½ teaspoon of dried oregano
- Salt and ground black pepper, as required
- 4 (5-ounce of) skinless, boneless chicken breasts, butterflied and pounded

Instructions:

1. Preheat your oven to 350 degrees F.
2. Line a baking sheet with parchment paper.

3. In a saucepan, heat the vegetable oil over medium heat and sauté onion and both peppers for about 1 minute.

4. Add the garlic and spinach and cook for about 2-3 minutes or until just wilted.

5. Stir in oregano, salt, and black pepper, and take away the saucepan from heat.

6. Place the chicken mixture into the center of every butterflied chicken breast.

7. Fold each chicken breast over filling to form a touch pocket and secure with toothpicks.

8. Arrange the chicken breasts onto the prepared baking sheet.

9. Bake for about 18-20 minutes.

10. Serve warm.

Balsamic Chicken Breast

Servings: 4

Preparation Time: 10 minutes

Cooking Time: 14 minutes

Ingredients:

- ¼ cup of balsamic vinegar
- 2 tablespoons of olive oil
- 1½ teaspoons of fresh lemon juice
- ½ teaspoon of lemon-pepper seasoning
- 4 (6-ounce of) boneless, skinless chicken breast halves, pounded slightly
- 6 cups of fresh baby kale

Instructions:

1. In a glass baking dish, place the vinegar, oil, juice, and seasoning and blend well.
2. Add the chicken breasts and coat with the mixture generously.
3. Refrigerate to marinate for about 25-30 minutes.
4. Preheat the grill to medium heat.

5. Grease the grill grate.

6. Remove the chicken from the bowl and discard the remaining marinade.

7. Place the chicken breasts onto the grill and canopy with the lid.

8. Cook for about 5-7 minutes per side or until desired doneness.

9. Serve hot alongside the kale.

Lemony Chicken Thighs

Servings: 4

Preparation Time: 10 minutes

Cooking Time: 16 minutes

Ingredients:

- 2 tablespoon of olive oil, divided
- 1 tablespoon of fresh lemon juice
- 1 tablespoon of lemon zest, grated
- 2 teaspoons of dried oregano
- 1 teaspoon of dried thyme
- Salt and ground black pepper, to taste
- 1½ pounds bone-in chicken thighs
- 6 cups of fresh baby spinach

Instructions:

1. Preheat your oven to 420 degrees F.
2. Add 1 tablespoon of the oil, lemon juice, lemon peel, dried herbs, salt, and black pepper in a large bowl and blend well.

3. Add the chicken thighs and coat with the mixture generously.

4. Refrigerate to marinate for at least 20 minutes.

5. In an oven-proof wok, heat the remaining oil over medium-high heat and sear the chicken thighs for about 2–3 minutes per side.

6. Immediately transfer the wok into the oven and Bake for about 10 minutes.

7. Serve hot alongside the spinach.

Spicy Chicken Drumsticks

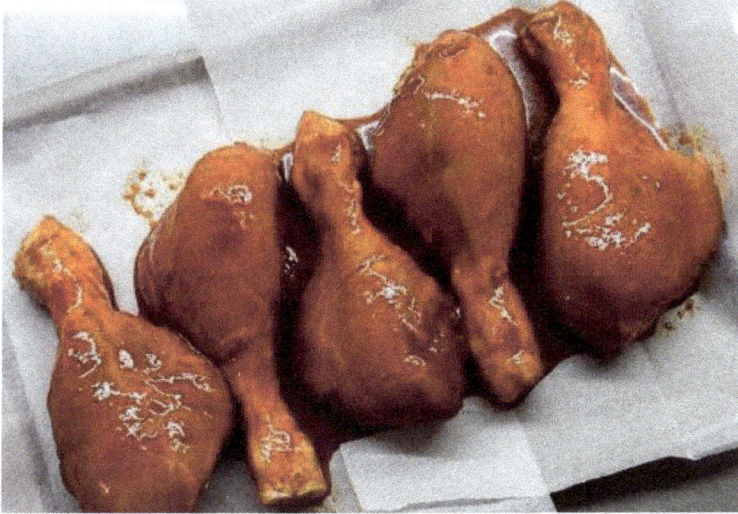

Servings: 5

Preparation Time: 10 minutes

Cooking Time: 40 minutes

Ingredients:

- 2 tablespoons of avocado oil
- 1 tablespoon of fresh lime juice
- 1 teaspoon of red chili powder
- 1 teaspoon of garlic powder
- Salt, as required

- 5 (8-ounce of) chicken drumsticks
- 8 cups of fresh baby arugula

Instructions:

1. In a bowl, mix avocado oil, lemon juice, chili powder, and garlic powder and blend well.
2. Add the chicken drumsticks and coat with the marinade generously.
3. Cover the bowl and refrigerate to marinate for about 30-60 minutes.
4. Preheat your grill to medium-high heat.
5. Place the chicken drumsticks onto the grill and cook for about 30-40 minutes, flipping after every 5 minutes.
6. Serve hot alongside the arugula.

Baked Chicken & Bell Peppers

Servings: 4

Preparation Time: 15 minutes

Cooking Time: 25 minutes

Ingredients:

- 1-pound boneless, skinless chicken breasts, cut into thin strips
- ½ of green bell pepper, seeded and cut into strips
- ½ of red bell pepper, seeded and cut into strips
- 1 medium onion, sliced
- 2 tablespoons of olive oil
- ½ teaspoon of dried oregano
- 2 teaspoons of chili powder
- 1½ teaspoons of ground cumin
- 1 teaspoon of garlic powder
- Salt, to taste

Instructions:

1. Preheat your oven to 400 degrees F.
2. In a bowl, add all the ingredients and blend well.

3. Place the chicken mixture into a 9x13-inch baking dish and spread it in a good layer.

4. Bake for about 20-25 minutes or until the chicken is completely baked.

5. Serve hot.

Orange Chicken

Servings: 6

Preparation Time: 10 minutes

Cooking Time: 20 minutes

Ingredients:

- 3 garlic cloves, minced
- ½ cup of fresh orange juice
- 1 tablespoon of apple cider vinegar
- 2 tablespoons of low-sodium soy sauce
- ¼ teaspoon of ground ginger
- ¼ teaspoon of ground cinnamon
- Freshly ground black pepper, to taste
- 2 pounds skinless, bone-in chicken thighs
- 1/3 cup of scallion, sliced

Instructions:

1. For marinating in a large bowl, mix together all ingredients apart from chicken thighs and scallion.
2. Add the chicken thighs and coat with marinade generously.

3. Cover the bowl and refrigerate to marinate for about 4 hours.

4. Remove the chicken from the bowl, reserving marinade.

5. Heat a lightly greased large non-stick skillet over medium-high heat and cook the chicken thighs for about 5-6 minutes or till golden brown.

6. Flip the side and cook for about 4 minutes.

7. Stir in the reserved marinade and bring to a boil.

8. Reduce the heat to medium-low and cook, covered for about 6-8 minutes or until sauce becomes thick.

9. Stir in the scallion and take away from the heat.

10. Serve hot

Chicken Breast with Asparagus

Servings: 5

Preparation Time: 15 minutes

Cooking Time: 16 minutes

Ingredients:

For Chicken:

- ¼ cup of extra-virgin olive oil
- ¼ cup of fresh lemon juice
- 2 tablespoons of maple syrup
- 1 garlic clove, minced
- Salt and ground black pepper, as required
- 5 (6-ounce of) boneless, skinless chicken breasts

For Asparagus:

- 1½ pounds of fresh asparagus
- 2 tablespoons of extra-virgin olive oil

Instructions:

1. For marinade: In a large bowl, add oil, lemon juice, Erythritol, garlic, salt, and black pepper, and beat until well combined.

2. In a large resealable bag, place the chicken and ¾ cup of marinade.

3. Seal the bag and shake to coat well.

4. Refrigerate overnight.

5. Cover the bowl of remaining marinade and refrigerate before serving.

6. Preheat the grill to medium heat. Grease the grill grate.

7. Remove the chicken from the bag and discard the marinade.

8. Place the chicken onto grill grate and grill, covered for about 5-8 minutes per side.

9. Meanwhile, in a pan of boiling water, arrange a steamer basket.

10. Place the asparagus in a steamer basket and steam, covered for about 5-7 minutes.

11. Drain the asparagus well and transfer into a bowl.

12. Add oil and toss to coat well.

13. Divide the chicken breasts and asparagus onto serving plates and serve.

Chicken with Zoodles

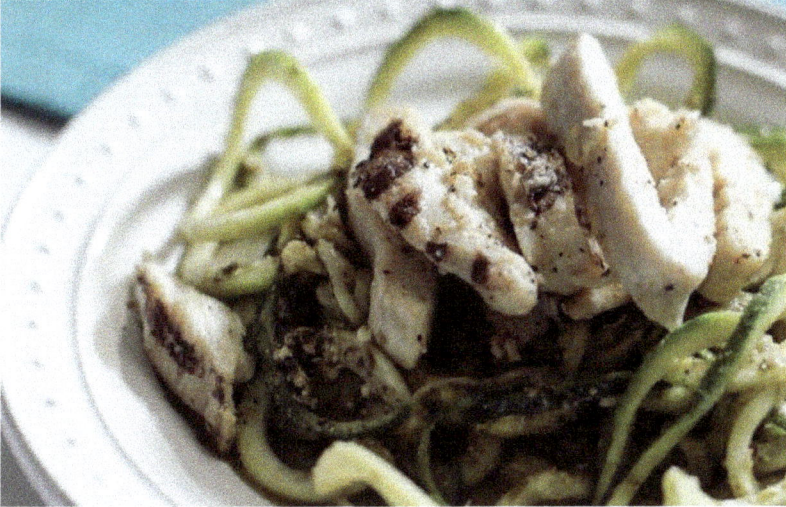

Servings: 4

Preparation Time: 15 minutes

Cooking Time: 18 minutes

Ingredients:

- 2 cups of zucchini, spiralized with Blade
- Salt, to taste
- 1½ pounds boneless, skinless chicken breasts
- Freshly ground black pepper, to taste
- 1 tablespoon of olive oil

- 1 cup of low-fat plain Greek yogurt
- ¼ cup of low-fat Parmesan cheese, shredded
- ½ cup of low-sodium chicken broth
- ½ teaspoon of Italian seasoning
- ½ teaspoon of garlic powder
- 1 cup of fresh spinach, chopped
- 3-6 slices of sun-dried tomatoes
- 1 tablespoon of garlic, chopped

Instructions:

1. Preheat your oven to 350 degrees F.
2. Line a large baking sheet with parchment paper.
3. Place the zucchini noodles and salt onto the prepared baking sheet and toss to coat well.
4. Arrange the zucchini noodles in a good layer and Bake for about 15 minutes.
5. Meanwhile, season the chicken breasts with salt and black pepper.
6. In a large skillet, heat the oil over medium-high heat and cook the chicken breasts for about 4-5 minutes per side or until cooked through.
7. With a slotted spoon, transfer the cooked chicken onto a plate and put aside.

8. In the same skillet, add the yogurt, Parmesan cheese, broth, Italian seasoning, and garlic powder and beat until well combined.

9. Place the skillet over medium-high heat and cook for about 2-3 minutes or until it starts to thicken, stirring continuously.

10. Stir in the spinach, sun-dried tomatoes, and garlic and cook for about 2-3 minutes.

11. Add the chicken breasts and cook for about 1-2 minutes.

12. Divide the zucchini noodles onto serving plates and top each with chicken mixture.

13. Serve immediately.

Chicken with Yellow Squash

Servings: 6

Preparation Time: 15 minutes

Cooking Time: 17 minutes

Ingredients:

- 2 tablespoons of olive oil, divided
- 1½ pounds skinless, boneless chicken breasts, cut into bite-sized pieces
- Salt and freshly ground black pepper, to taste
- 2 garlic cloves, minced
- 1½ pounds yellow squash, sliced
- 2 tablespoons of fresh lemon juice
- 1 teaspoon of fresh lemon zest, grated finely
- 2 tablespoons of fresh parsley, minced

Instructions:

1. In a large skillet, heat 1 tablespoon of oil over medium heat and fry chicken for about 6-8 minutes or until golden brown from all sides.
2. Transfer the chicken onto a plate.

3. In the same skillet, heat remaining oil over medium heat and sauté garlic for about 1 minute.
4. Add the squash slices and cook for about 5-6 minutes,
5. Stir in the chicken and cook for about 2 minutes.
6. Stir in the lemon juice, zest, and parsley and take away from heat.
7. Serve hot.